Essential oils:
Top 30 proven essential oil recipes for instant pain relief!

Table of content

Introduction

Essential oils have been used for over thousands of years. They have been proven successful both in the scientific life as well as for amazing use in homes. Essential oils contain extractions from some useful plants, and from many parts of a plant. When essential oil was first discovered, the Egyptians and the Jews used to soak the plants in the oil and then used to take the oil by straining it.

Essential oils have amazing anti inflammation properties, protect against bacteria and they are very amazing anti oxidants. Essential oils can be used to serve numerous purposes such as window cleaners, fabric softeners, mosquito repellants, body washes, soaps, baby wipes, foot scrubs, as detergents, air refreshers and even in drinks, some of which are mentioned later in this book.

There are a few methods for the extraction of essential oils, namely distillation, expression, and solvent extraction. In the process of distillation, parts of the plants such as the leaves, flowers, stems barks and all are placed in the distillation can over water. As the water is steamed, the steam goes down the parts of the plant making the parts soft, extracting their oil and then the vapor passes through and is collected in the vessel. The vapor is cooled and condenses into liquid and that makes the essential oil.

In expression the citrus fruits are used such as oranges and lemons. Their skins are peeled off and then used to make the essential oil. These essential oils of the citrus fruits are generally much cheaper than the other essential oils available. The process involved in the citrus fruits is somewhat similar to that of extracting the olive oil. They normally are expressed to get the essential oil or cold pressed which is similar to the extraction of olive oil.

An alternate process of extracting the essential oil apart from distillation is known as the solvent extraction. This process was found because some parts of the plant specially the flowers were found to be very delicate and lost their power when gone through the process of distillation because of the high heat in distillation. Apart from hexane, carbondioxide is also used as a solvent in the extraction of essential oils.

Essential oils are widely used in pharmacies, and are considered to be of good use in medicines and for health purposes. They are also used in aromatherapy, which is for healing effects. They are also used to solve allergy conditions, irritated and itchy skin also.

Therefore, it can be seen that essential oils serve a wide variety of purposes and are really beneficial for human beings. They have a lot of natural ingredients in them and can be used in our day to lives. For your own benefit, it is a healthy choice to select a few essential oils and keep at your home for your use. You will find ahead almost 25 proven recipes of how essential oils can be used in your lives!

Chapter 01: essential oil recipes for treatment of sore joints, muscles and pain

1. ACHES, PAIN, RHEUMATISM

Description: This essential oil recipe is to treat pains associated with either menstrual pains or cramps following a vigorous exercise or back aches or any kind of other aches. It is a helpful and easy recipe.

Ingredients:

- Ten drops of rosemary

- Six drops of juniper berry

- Eight drops of lavender

- 45 ml of any oil

Recipe: Take a jar and add in the drops of rosemary, juniper berry, lavender drops and any oil of your choice. Combine all the oils and then apply them where ever you feel you have pain.

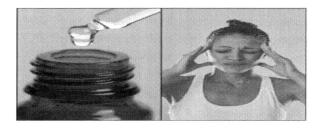

2. MASSAGE OIL FOR SORE MUSCLES

Introduction: This recipe of essential oil is for those who have sore muscles. Soreness of the muscles can be caused by either heavy exercise, due to age factor or a very tiring schedule. The following is the recipe of an essential oil which will help you to cure this problem.

Ingredients:

- Two drops of ginger

- Four drops of cinnamon

- Three drops of cajuput

- Three drops of chamomile

- 15 to 20 ml of any of your choice of oil

Recipe: In a jar mix in the ginger, cinnamon, cajuput, chamomile and your choice of oil and mix properly all kinds of oils until all are combined. Apply this oil on to your muscles specially after a full day workout.

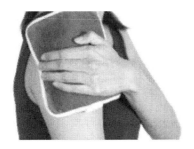

3. ESSENTIAL OIL FOR SORE JOINTS

Description : This recipe of essential oil is particularly handy for those who have severe pain the joints. It is recommended for old people who face this problem often. Below is the recipe of it.

Ingredients:

- 10 drops of marjoram

- 8 drops of eucalyptus

- Four drops of cajuput

- 2 drops of black pepper

- One cup of carrier oil

Recipe: In a jar, mix the marjoram, eucalyptus, cajuput and the drops of black pepper. Shake well and then add in the carrier oil. Mix until everything is combined. Apply on effected areas and sore joints.

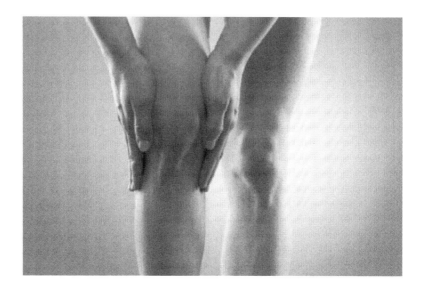

4. ESSENTIAL OIL FOR BACH ACHE MASSAGE

Description: The problem of back ache is very common specially among women as they have a tiring schedule all day and when they have responsibilities of kids. Back aches are found in men too who have the job of driving all day or to sit on uncomfortable office chairs. Below is the recipe of the essential oil to cure back aches.

Ingredients:

- Two tablespoons of almond oil

- Ten drops of lavender

- Six drops of rosemary

- Six drops of sandalwood

- Three drops of geranium

Recipe: Take an amber bottle, and add in the almond oil, the lavender, rosemary, sandalwood and the geranium and shake until all the ingredients are properly mixed. Apply to your back and massage or ask your companion to massage on your back.

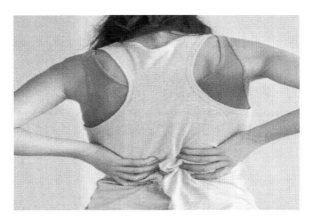

5. ESSENTIAL OILS FOR ACHING MUSCLES

Description: Muscles tend to ache either because of age factor, weakness, un balanced diet, poor nutrition and many other factors. For that we provide you with an easy and natural recipe of essential oil to cure it. Below is the recipe of it.

Ingredients:

- Four drops of peppermint

- Four drops of thyme

- Four drops of lavender

- Three drops of marjoram

- Carrier oil any of your choice, 5 ml

Recipe: In a jar, mix the peppermint essential oil, the thyme, lavender and the marjoram. Then add in the carrier oil and mix properly and apply to the affected areas. This essential oil can also be used in the bath tub but only for those who do not have allergy from peppermint essential oil.

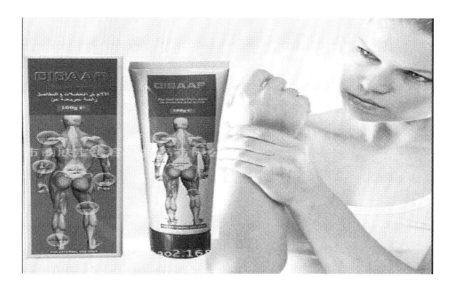

Chapter 02: essential oil recipes for burns

6. EMERGENCY BURN COMPRESS OR WASH

Description: A burn on our skins can be very painful and difficult to handle. This recipe of essential oil burn compress provides quick relief from burns. Below is the recipe of it.

Ingredients:

- One pint of water at a temperature of 50 degrees Fahrenheit

- Five drops of lavender oil

Recipe: Add the lavender oil in to the water as to properly mix in the oil with water. With a help of a soft cloth or towel dip the cloth in to the liquid and let it soak for about 10 minutes. Put the cloth on the burnt area for a while and then remove. You can also soak the burnt area in the oil to get relief.

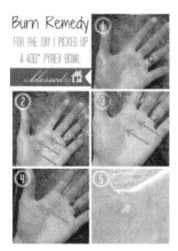

7. AFTER BURN ESSENTIAL OIL FORMULA

Description: Instead of using the tubes available in the market at such expensive rates it is better to apply essential oil to the burnt area. Here we provide you with a recipe of essential oil for the treatment of burns.

Ingredients:

- Two drops of peppermint essential oil

- 25 drops of lavender essential oil

- Two ounces of sunflower oil

Recipe: Mix in the peppermint essential oil, the lavender essential oil and the sunflower oil. Mix all the oils and then apply on the affected area two to three times a day. It will cure in no time.

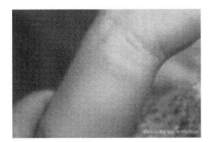

8. LAVENDAR AND ALOE VERA ESSENTIAL OIL RECIPE

Description: Lavender and aloe vera have many useful qualities. Apart from their smell they are pretty useful in other stuff. For example in the treatment of burns both lavender and aloevera play an important role. Below is the recipe of such essential oil.

Ingredients:

- Twenty drops of lavender essential oil

- One cup of fresh aloe vera gel

Recipe: Mix the lavender essential oil and the fresh aloe vera gel and they both combine to be an excellent healing agent. Apply to the affected area and cover the wound with a dressing. It will heal in no time. Change the dressing two times a day or more depending upon the severity of the condition.

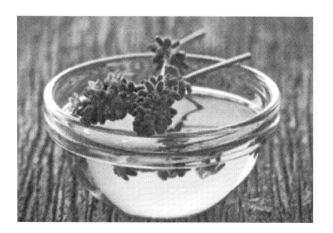

9. HOME MADE BURN FORMULA

Description: This recipe of essential oil is very easy and quick to make at home. It is recommended to make it and store it to use in emergency conditions. Below is the recipe of it.

Ingredients:

- Eight drops of lavender essential oil or five drops of roman chamomile oil
- One bowl of cold water

Recipe: Mix the cold water and the lavender or chamomile oil until the oil is properly diffused with the water. You can add ice cubes to make the water colder. Dip the burnt area in to this oil for immense relief. You can also take a cloth, dip in the oil and then apply the cloth on to your burnt skin.

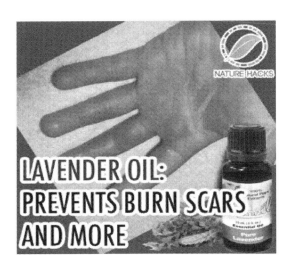

10. ESSENTIAL OIL BLEND FOR SUN BURNS

Description : People go out on the beach to enjoy and to relax. Sometimes the heat of the sun is so severe that instead of getting a tan we get sun burns which are very irritating and sometimes very painful as well. Below you will find a recipe of a comforting blend to cure sun burns.

Ingredients:

- One tub of cool water

- One drop of pepper mint

- Two drops of helichrysum

- two drops of roman chamomile

- eight drops of lavender essential oil

Recipe: In a tub of cool water, add in the pepper mint, helichrysum, roman chamomile and the lavender essential oil and mix. Apply this mixture on to the affected sunburn and let it soak for about 15 minutes. Do this twice or thrice a day to get complete relief.

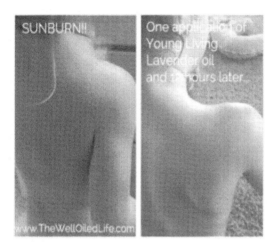

11. SOOTHING BLEND TO CURE BURNS

Description: This essential oil is to cure and sooth the burns on the skin which cause real pain. It is fairly easy and quick to make with only a few ingredients. Below is the recipe of it.

Ingredients:

- twenty drops of lavender essential oil

- five teaspoons of fresh aloe vera juice

- one teaspoon of sea buckthorn oil

Recipe: Take a glass container of one ounce and add in the lavender essential oil, aloe vera juice and the sea buckthorn oil and mix. Before using shake the bottle and with the help of a cotton ball apply the oil very gently and carefully to the affected area.

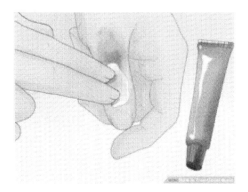

12. ESSENTIAL OIL RECIPE TO MEND SCARS

Description: This recipe of essential oil is made to mend scars on the skin. Sometimes the scars on the skin can cause real irritation and problems. For this we have provided you with a recipe of essential oil. Below is the recipe of it.

Ingredients:

- two ounces of grape seed oil

- five drops of tea tree oil

- five drops of lavender oil

Recipe: Take a glass container and add in the grape seed oil, the tea tree oil and the lavender oil and mix properly. Let sit the oil for a day or two before applying it on your scars. Apply twice a day.

Chapter 03: essential oil recipes to fight cold and flu

13. PROTECTIVE OIL BLEND

Description: This protective oil blend recipe of essential oil used to treat cold and flu problems. It is a very handy oil which is made from natural ingredients. Below is the recipe of it.

Ingredients:

- twenty drops of clove oil
- 18 drops of lemon oil
- Ten drops of cinnamon bark oil
- Eight drops of eucalyptus oil
- Five drops of rosemary oil

Recipe: In a dark glass container, add in the clove oil, the lemon oil, the cinnamon bark oil, the eucalyptus oil and the rosemary oil and mix it well. Use it when you have flu or cold. This oil can also be used to purify the air, and as a disinfectant.

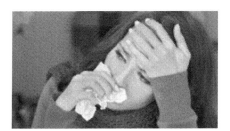

14. ESSENTIAL OIL TO TREAT COUGH

Description: This recipe of essential oil is amazing for those who want to treat their cough and congestion problems naturally rather than treat it with the chemical stuffed syrups and tablets available out there. Below is the recipe of it.

Ingredients:

- Few drops of Cyprus

- 3 drops of pepper mint essential oil

- eucalyptus oil

Recipe : Drop the Cyprus, peppermint and the eucalyptus oil together under your pillow before sleeping in the night and sleep on your pillow. This help to reduce your cough when you are trying to sleep in the night and make your sleep to be restful and peace.

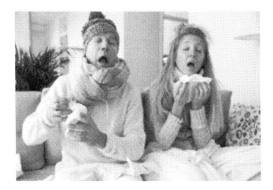

Description: The vapo rubs and chest rubs available in the market are full of chemicals and harmful substances. Instead of using them we provide you with an easy and natural recipe of a home made chest rub using essential oils. Below is the recipe of it.

Ingredients:

- $1/4^{th}$ ounce of organic beeswax

- $1/4^{th}$ cup of organic coconut oil

- Ten drops of eucalyptus essential oil

- Ten drops of peppermint essential oil

- Ten drops of fir needle essential oil or wintergreen essential oil

Recipe: In a double boiler melt the coconut oil and the bees wax until both are incorporated together. Remove from heat and let them cool slightly. Now add in the eucalyptus essential oil, the peppermint essential oil and the fir needle essential oil and mix everything together. Store this oil in a glass container and apply to the soles of feet and chest to avoid cold getting you.

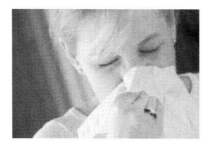

16. MICROBIAL STEAM INHALATION ESSENTIAL OIL

Description: This microbial steam inhalation essential oil is for those who get cold and flu very frequently. It is very helpful to cure cold problems very quickly. This recipe is very easy and fairly quick to make. Following is the recipe.

Ingredients:

- 2 drops of thyme
- Two drops of sage
- 2 drops of lavender
- 2 drops of lemon grass
- Few drops of grape fruit
- One bowl of warm water

Recipe: In a steaming bowl of warm water add in the few drops of thyme, sage, lavender, lemon grass and the grape fruit and mix everything properly. Bring your face closer to this steaming bowl of the essential oil and try to inhale deeply the steam coming out from it. Make sure to not come in direct contact with the water. Breath in for few minutes to clear the blocked passages of your nose.

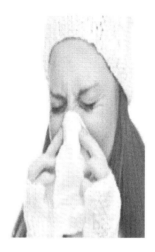

17. GERM FIGHTING SPRITZER FOR ALLERGIES

Description: This essential oil spritzer is made to avoid cold and flu problems caused because of allergies in the environment. It is made with few ingredients and is very helpful to solve the problem of fighting germs. Below is the recipe of it.

Ingredients:

- 1 ¾ ounces of water

- 10 to 30 drops of different essential oils such as lavender essential oil, eucalyptus essential oil, cinnamon essential oil.

- A quarter of a teaspoon of witch hazel to mix in the oil and water

Recipe: In a 2 ounce container fill in the water, witch hazel, the lavender essential oil, cinnamon essential oil and the eucalyptus essential oil and shake to mix everything well. You can keep this bottle at your home, at office or even in your pocket for instant use.

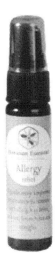

Chapter 04: essential oil recipes for the treatment of headaches

18. ESSENTIAL OIL RECIPES TO TREAT HEADACHES BECAUSE OF LOW BLOOD SUGAR LEVELS

Description: This kind of head ache is known as the sugar head ache because it is caused when a person has low blood sugar level in their body. A recipe of an essential oil is provided for you to solve this problem, below is the recipe.

Ingredients:

- One tablespoon of coconut oil
- One tablespoon of lavender essential oil
- One tablespoon of rosemary
- One drop of rosemary

Recipe: Combine equal amounts of lavender essential oil, the coconut oil and the rosemary and apply this mixture on the back of your neck or temples and on your forehead. Another alternative way of using this recipe is by adding one drop of rosemary to any smoothie you have and drink it.

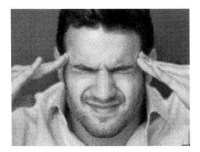

19. BASIC HEADACHE MASSAGE RECIPE

Description: This recipe of essential oil is the most basic recipe of an aromatherapy massage essential oil. Using this recipe and massaging on the head can give you quick relief from the nasty headaches you get after a tiring day. Following is the recipe for it.

Ingredients:

- One ounce of carrier oil for instance jojoba oil or sweet almond oil

- Peppermint essential oil, 6 to 8 drops

- One ounce of an amber bottle or cobalt glass bottle

Recipe: In your bottle of either the amber or the cobalt mix in your choice of carrier oil (jojoba or sweet almond oil) and add in the peppermint essential oil. Instead of pepper mint essential oil you can also use eucalyptus essential oil. Mix the bottle with the lid on tight and shake so that the oil is mixed properly.

When you want to use, put one to four drops on the palms of your hands and apply and massage on your forehead or temples or on your neck. To avoid any mishap it is advised to keep the oil away from your eyes.

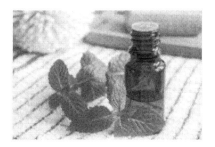

20. TISSUE AND COTTON BALL DIFFUSION RECIPE FOR HEAD ACHES

Description: Headaches can be really disturbing and can cause a real hindrance in ones work and a great deal of delay also. It is necessary to cure them as soon as possible to stay calm and fit. For this we provide you with a very easy recipe for the treatment of headaches using essential oils.

Ingredients:

- A cotton ball or a tissue

- Lavender essential oil

- Spearmint essential oil

Recipe: Using either the cotton ball or a tissue, whenever you get a head ache that really irritates you put a few drops of the lavender essential oil and the spearmint essential oil and then inhale through your nose. For beginners it is recommended to put only one drop on the tissue as to check if the person has allergy or not. The headache will cure using this method.

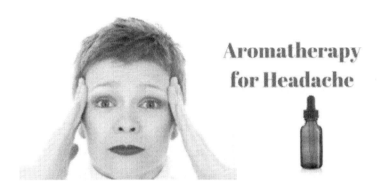

21. ESSENTIAL OIL RECIPE FOR TENSION HEADACHES

Description: This kind of headache is associated with taking pressure and are known as stress headaches. Some people are prone to taking a lot of stress and tension, over thinking stuff a lot. It is not a good thing and can lead to severe headaches. Following is the recipe using essential oils to cure these kind of headaches.

Ingredients:

- Warm water bath

- Five to ten drops of lavender essential oil

Recipe: When having a severe head ache, a hot water bath is recommended to ease the pain. Put the lavender essential oil in the hot water bath and take a bath to let the pressure and stress reduce. It is also recommended to apply pepper mint oil on the neck or on the temples to reduce the pain.

www.humblebeeandme.com

Make your own
Essential Oil
Headache Eraser

22. ESSENTIAL OIL RECIPE TO CURE MIGRAINE HEADACHES

Description: Migraine headaches have become really common in the recent times even in the young generation and causes a lot of disturbance in ones routine. It is particularly painful and difficult to ignore. Below we provide you with an easy way to cure migraine headaches using essential oils.

Ingredients:

- Few drops of lavender essential oil

- Few drops of pepper mint essential oil

Recipe: It is your choice to use either lavender essential oil or the pepper mint essential oil or either you can mix both. Apply these essential oils on your temples or neck to get rid of migraine and feelings of anxiety and nausea because of the migraine.

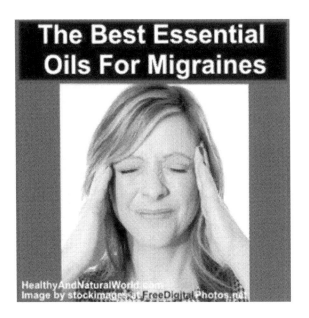

23. MIGRAINE RELIEF ESSENTIAL OIL RECIPE

Description : Migraines can be really painful, and instead of having chemically stuffed tablets or antibiotics who have no healthy value it is better to cure this problem using essential oils. Below is the recipe for the treatment of migraine using essential oils.

Ingredients:

- one drop of frankincense

- two drops of peppermint essential oil

- M grain 3 drops

Recipe: These are some multiple essential oils which can be used differently for the treatment of migraines. For frankincense it is advised to use one drop only on the roof of the mouth.

For peppermint essential oil it is advised to put the drops on the temple and massage gently.

For m grain it is advised to put the drops on the back of your neck and massage gently.

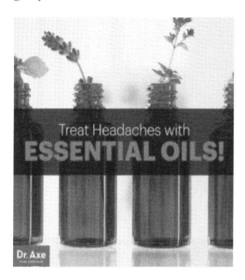

24. ROOM MISTS FOR HEADACHES USING ESSENTIAL OILS

Description: Some people get really allergic and irritated because of nasty and bad smells in the environment. They even get a bad headache because of the smell. For this, we have provided you with a mist recipe using essential oil. Below is the way to make it.

Ingredients:

- A four ounce clean spray bottle

- 30 to 40 drops of your choice of essential oil, preferably lavender essential oil because of its amazing fragrance

- 1.5 ounces of alcohol

Recipe: With the help of the spray bottle add in the distilled water and the lavender essential oil, now add the alcohol to mix properly and mix until everything is mixed properly. Spray whenever you feel sick and discomfort because of the smell in the environment.

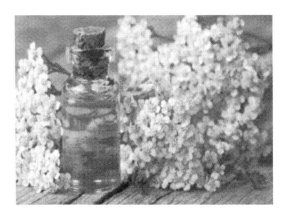

25. ROOM MIST RECIPE USING ESSENTIAL OILS

Description: This recipe of a room mist contains very fragrant essential oils which will make your room and environment smell very nice and fresh. Below is the recipe of it.

Ingredients:

- Twenty drops of rosemary essential oil

- Eight drops of grapefruit essential oil

- Four drops of peppermint essential oil

- Two drops of spearmint essential oil

- 1.5 ounces of alcohol

- A clean spray bottle

Recipe: Using the spray bottle, add in the alcohol and then the rosemary essential oil, the grapefruit essential oil, the peppermint essential oil and the spearmint essential oil and mix. Let the bottle rest for a few minutes before using. Spray when there is bad smell in the room which is giving you headache.

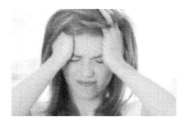

Chapter 05: essential oil recipes for peaceful sleep, calming kids and tension free life

25. ESSENTIAL OIL RECIPE FOR RELAXATION AND REJUVINATION

Description: Living happily and peacefully is a vital part of our lives. It is recommended by doctors also to live happily and to take care of our health. Health is wealth has always been heard. There are some essential oils which if used can be used to give relaxation after a tiring day. Following is the recipe of it.

Ingredients:

- Six drops of wintergreen

- Six drops of lavender

- Four drops of peppermint

- Four drops of frankincense

- Two drops of basil and rosemary

- Half cup of carrier oil

Recipe: Mix in the winter green essential oil, the lavender essential oil, the peppermint essential oil, the frankincense, the basil and the rosemary. Mix all the oils and now add in the carrier oil. Mix everything properly and then use it to relax and cherish every moment of your life in a peaceful environment.

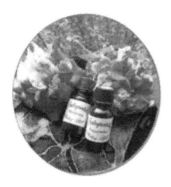

26. ESSENTIAL OIL RECIPE FOR PAIN RELIEF

Description : Essential oils can also be used for the treatment of pains. Pains can be of different kinds, they can either be in the joints, in the muscles, in the legs, thighs, hips or even backaches. A simple recipe can be used and made to cure them. Below is the recipe of it.

Ingredients:

- Eight drops of lavender
- Eight drops of lemon
- Four drops of marjoram
- Carrier oil half cup

Recipe: Mix in the carrier oil, and the lavender, the lemon and the marjoram and mix until completely mixed. The carrier oil can be either jojoba oil or coconut oil depending upon your choice. Apply this oil to the affected areas two or three times a day for quick results.

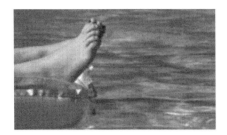

27. ESSENTIAL OIL RECIPE FOR A CALMING CHILD

Description: Babies are very cute and innocent until they cry that is. Babies can either make our world very wonderful or they can make our world full of anxiety and make us go mad by their crying and shrilling. This recipe using essential oils is for those babies who really need to be calm and composed. Below is the recipe of it.

Ingredients:

- Eighty drops of vetiver

- Thirty drops of lavender

- Thirty drops of ylang ylang

- Twenty drops of frankincense

- Fifteen drops of clary sage

- Ten drops of marjoram

- Thirty drops of coconut oil

Recipe: In a 10 ml of glass bottle, add in the coconut oil, the vetiver, the lavender essential oil. The ylang ylang, the frankincense, the clary sage and the marjoram and mix well until all the ingredients have been incorporated. Apply this oil to the soles of the feet or on the wrists of babies or on the palms.

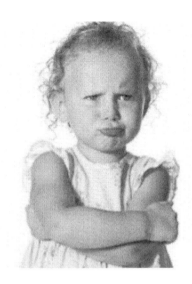

28. ESSENTIAL OIL RECIPE FOR UTTER CALMNESS

Description: A calm and composed nature, makes us to go very smoothly where as when a person is stressed too much can go wrong. Below we provide you with a recipe of essential oil to achieve extreme calmness.

Ingredients:

- Thirty drops of tangerine

- Thirty drops of orange

- Twenty drops of ylang ylang

- Ten drops of patchouli

- Four drops blue tansy

- Half cup of coconut oil

Recipe: Mix the tangerine, orange, ylang ylang, patchouli, blue tansy and the coconut oil. The coconut oil should only be added if you wish to do massage on your hair. This oil will help a great deal in making you extremely calm.

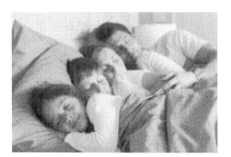

29. ESSENTIAL OIL FOR MENTAL CLARITY

Description: Essential oils are also used to achieve mental clarity and confidence. Below we provide with a recipe of such an essential oil.

Ingredients:

- Four drops of rosemary

- Six drops of lemon

- Two drops of cypress

Recipe: In a 10 ml bottle, mix in the rosemary, lemon and the cypress and shake well, apply to soles of feet or wrists or on the temples.

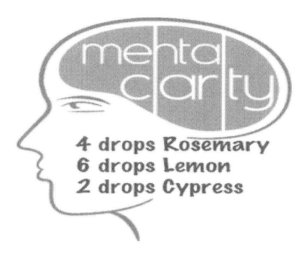

4 drops Rosemary
6 drops Lemon
2 drops Cypress

30. ESSENTIAL OIL RECIPE FOR PEACE AND CALM

Description: This recipe of essential oil is used to achieve peace and calmness. It is easy to make and contains few ingredients. Below is the recipe of it.

Ingredients:

- Twenty five drops of tangerine

- 25 drops of orange

- 15 drops of ylang ylang

- 10 drops of patchouli

- 4 drops of chamomile

   Recipe: Take a 5 ml bottle and add the tangerine, the orange, ylang ylang, patchouli and the chamomile and shake so that all the ingredients are mixed in properly. Apply to temples, wrists or soles of feet.

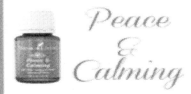

HOW TO MAKE YOUR OWN

Peace & Calming

SAVINGDOLLARSANDSENSE.COM

Conclusion

At the end of this e book, first I would like to thank all the readers, who took out their time and downloaded this e book. I am particularly thankful to all the readers out there. The advantages of essential oils have long been known, and to study them and the ingredients and the recipes which can be made using these essential oils can help you a great deal in your life.

This e book contains almost 30 valid and authentic recipes using essential oils as their core ingredient. Essential oils can be used to treat headaches, migraines, cold, congestion, flu, mental tiredness, sleep problems, anxiety problems, for calming babies and many many more.

By downloading this e book you can make sure that your life will be at a much better pace then it was ever before. Essential oils have a lot of advantages and the biggest advnantage this has is that it is much better to use these essential oil recipes which are natural rather than using tablets and medicines and tubes from the market which are not only harmful for the health but also uselessly expensive.

I hope that all of you had an amazing time reading this e book and would appreciate your comments on this e book. Feel free to ask any question or query you wish to ask. In the end I would like to wish each and every reader a happy reading! Adios!

FREE Bonus Reminder

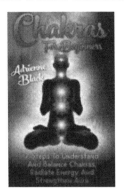

If you have not grabbed it yet, please go ahead and download your special bonus E book *"Chakras for Beginners. 7 Steps To Understand And Balance Chakras, Radiate Energy, And Strengthen Aura"*.

Simply Click the Button Below

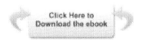

OR Go to This Page

http://lifehacksworld.com/free

BONUS #2: More Free & Discounted Books & Products

Do you want to receive more Free/Discounted Books or Products?

We have a mailing list where we send out our new Books or Products when they go free or with a discount on Amazon. Click on the link below to sign up for Free & Discount Book & Product Promotions.

=> Sign Up for Free & Discount Book & Product Promotions <=

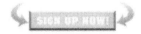

OR Go to this URL

http://zbit.ly/1WBb1Ek

Made in the USA
San Bernardino, CA
15 March 2017